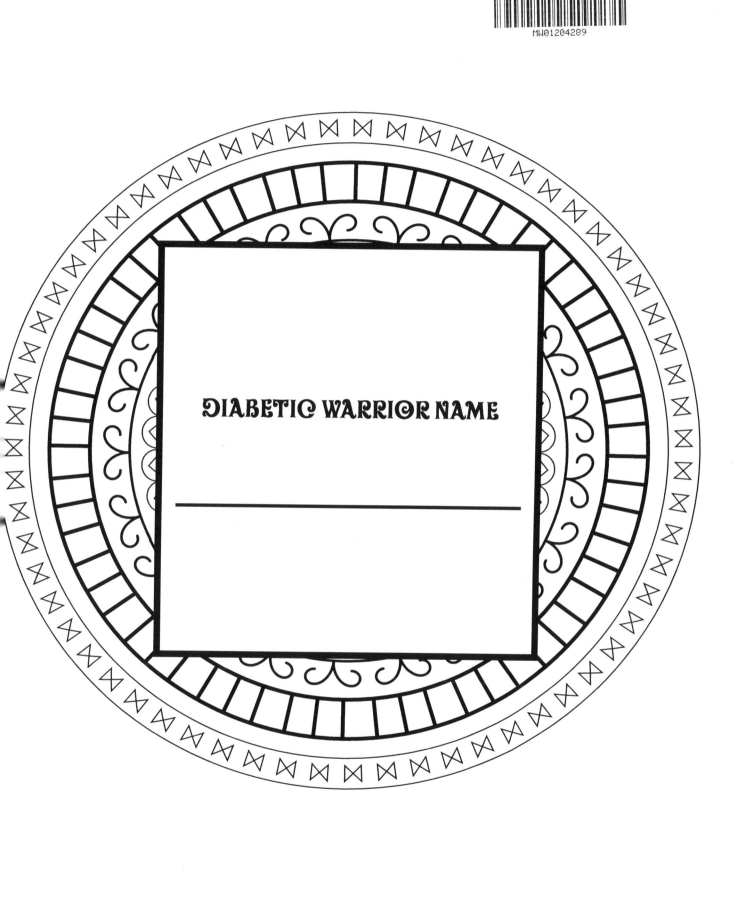

DIABETIC WARRIOR NAME

WE HOPE THIS COLORING BOOK BRINGS YOU JOY, HAPPINESS, AND A GOOD LAUGH. KEEP FIGHTING YOU BEAUTIFUL WARRIOR.

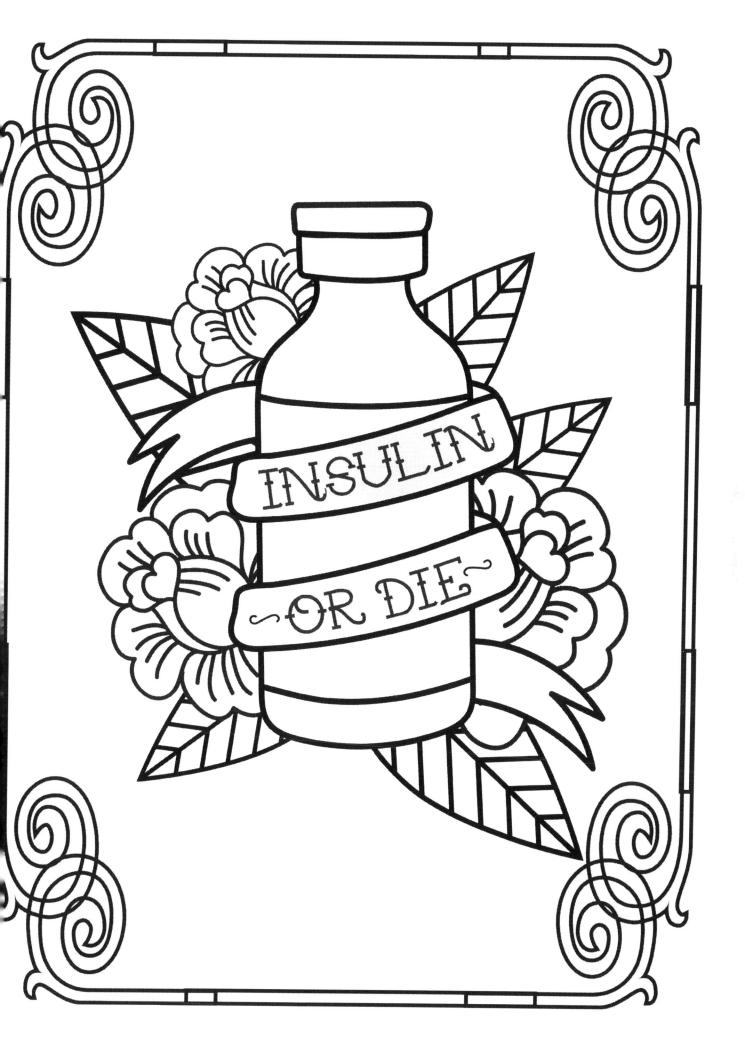

INSULIN OR DIE

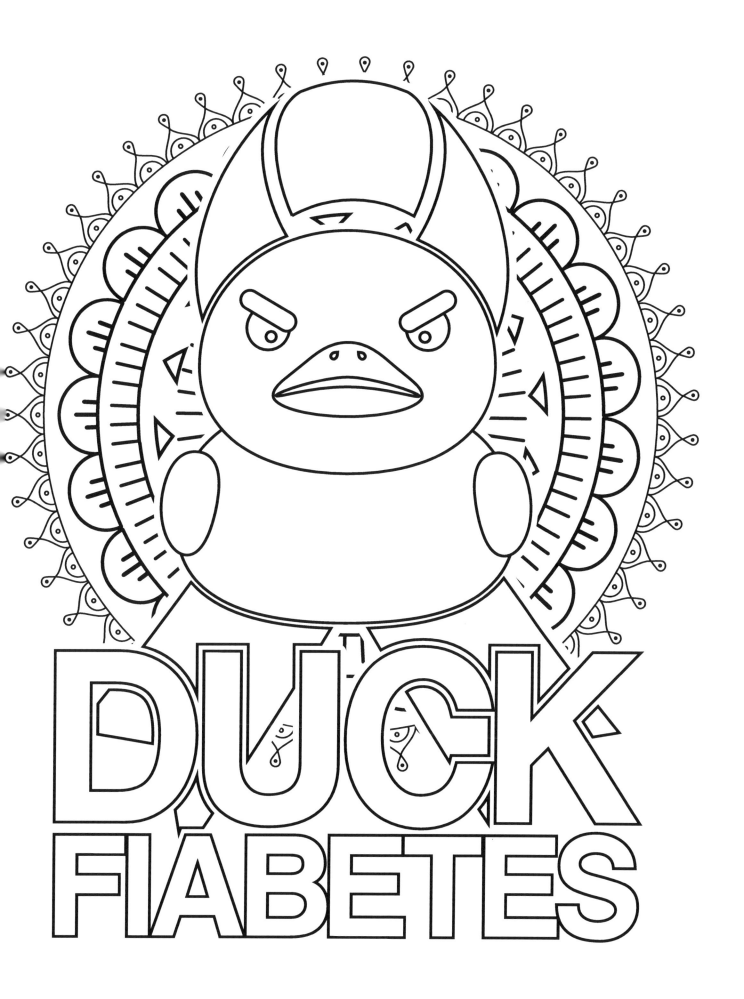

DUCK FIABETES

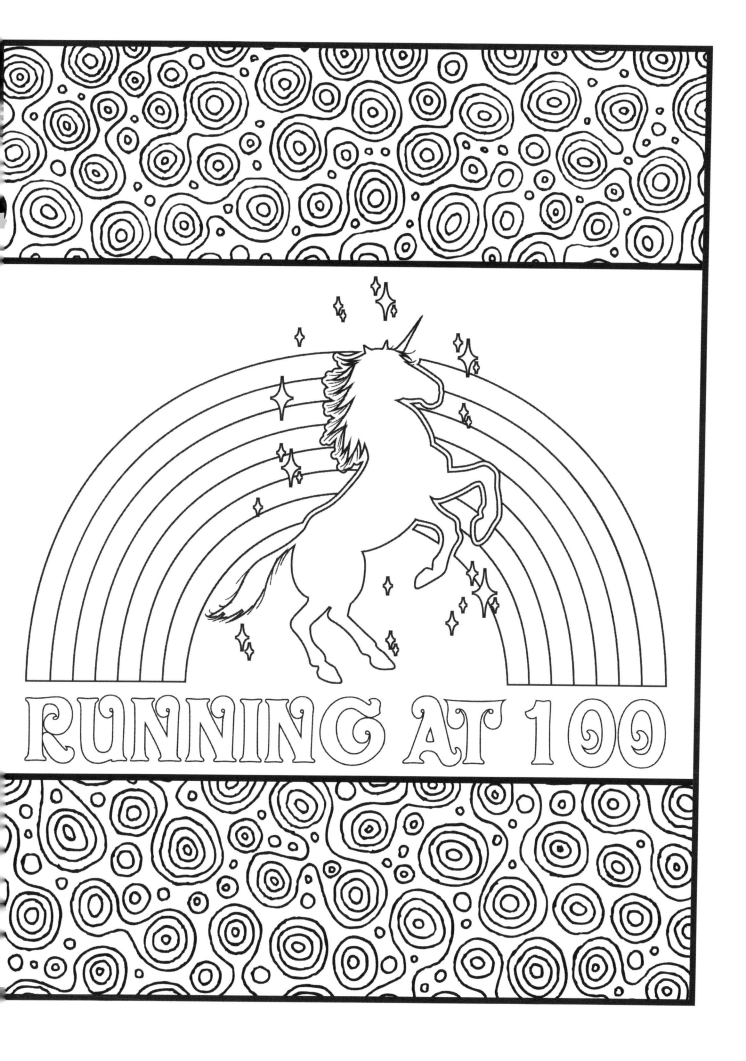

RUNNING AT 100

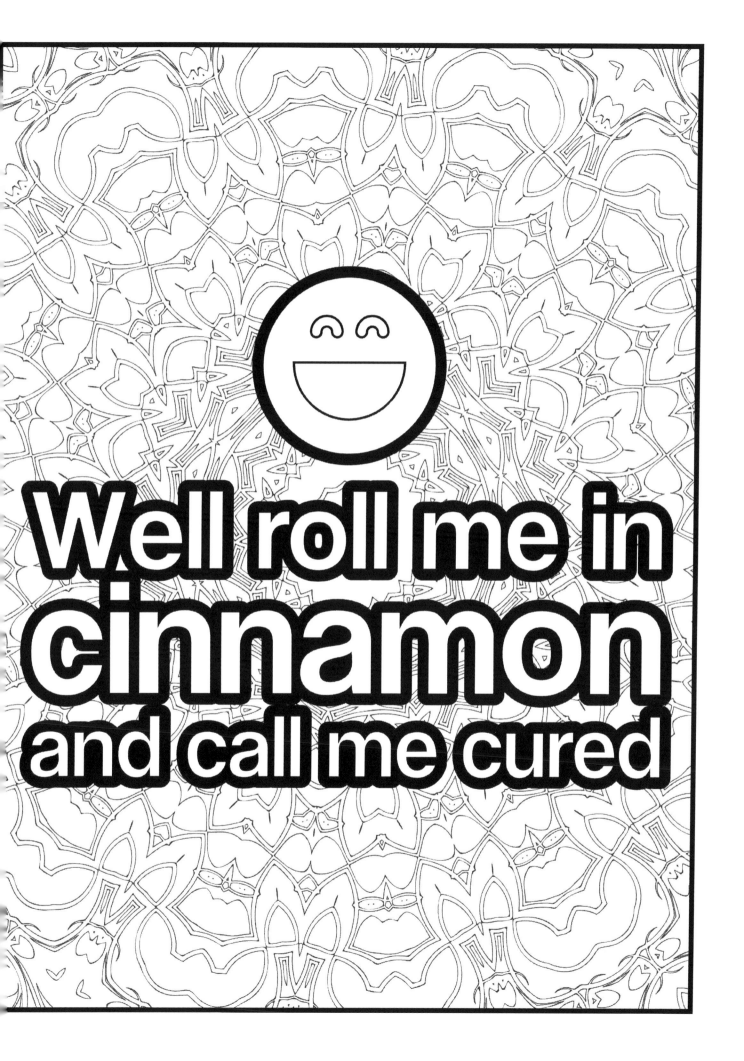

WELL CALL ME CURED

Juice Box Zombie

JUICE BOX ZOMBIE

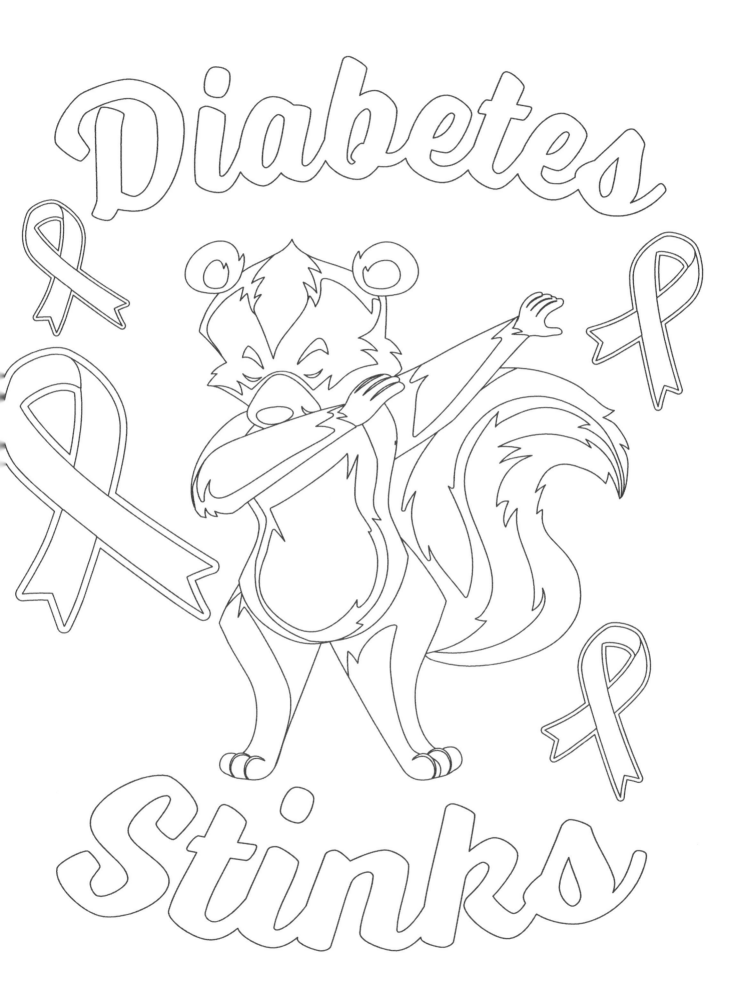

DIABETES STINKS

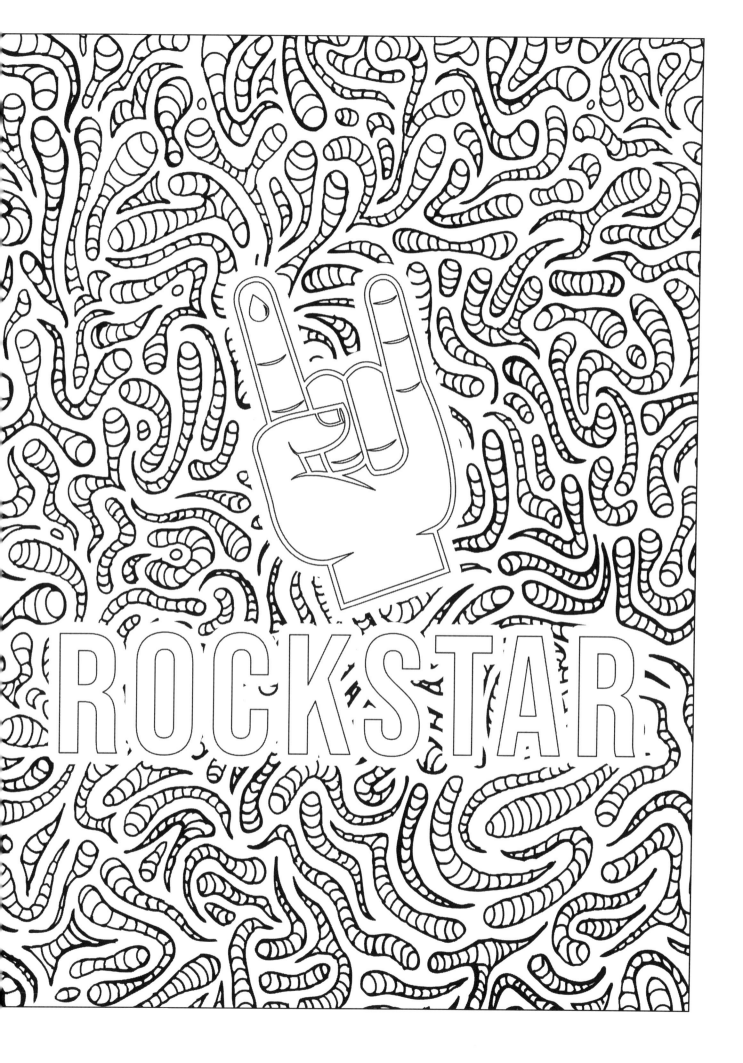

ROCKSTAR

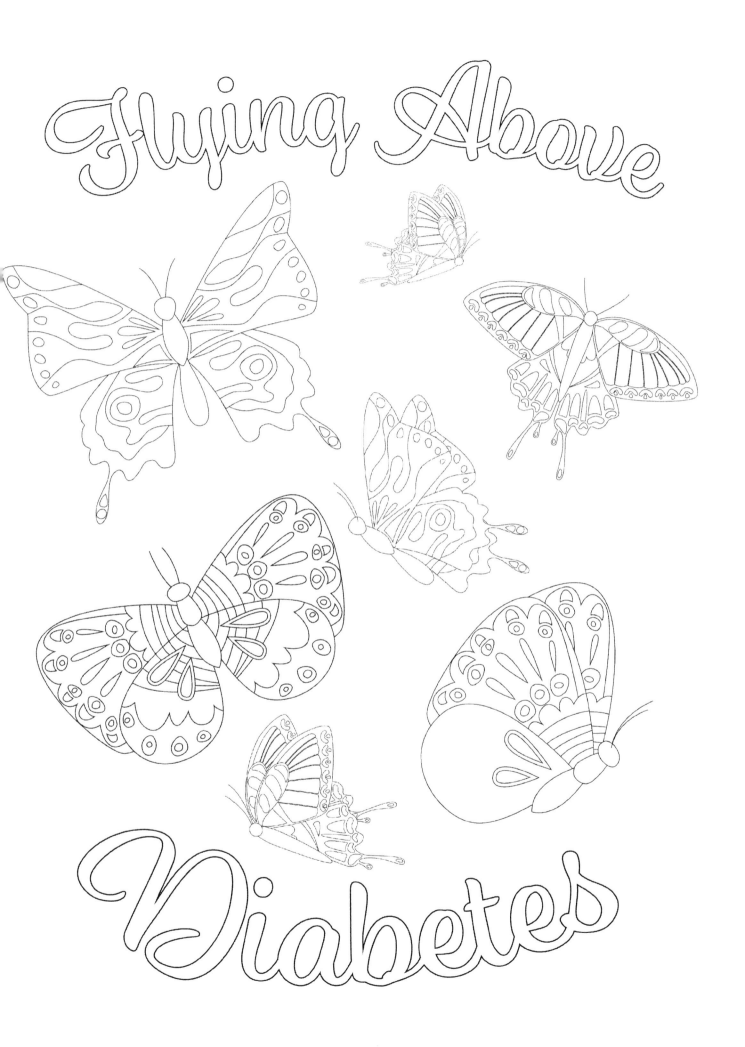

FLYING ABOVE DIABETES

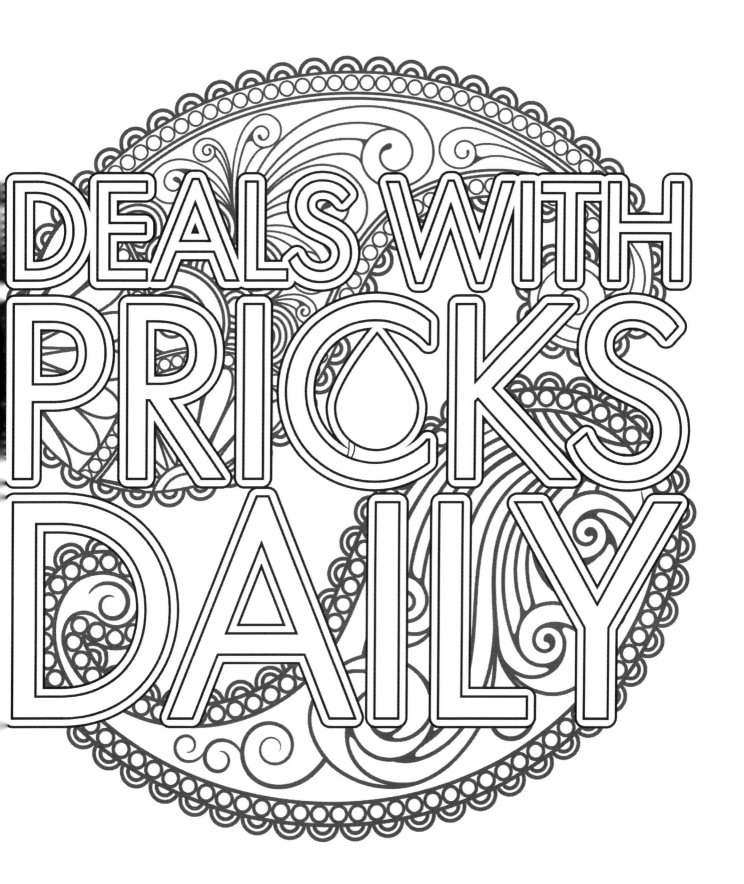

DEALS WITH PRICKS DAILY

Dreaming

Of A Cure

DREAMING OF A CURE

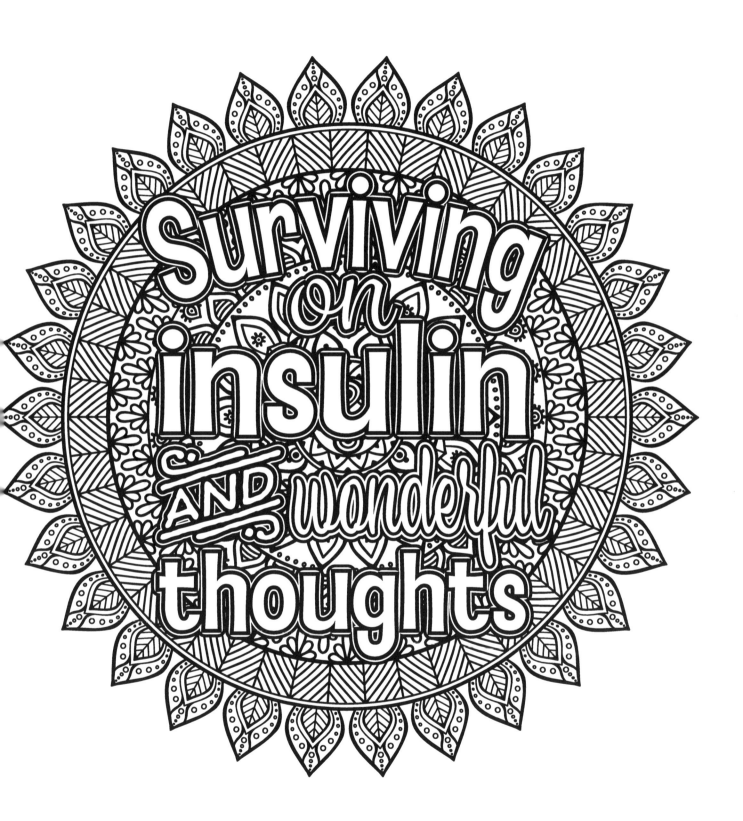

SURVIVING ON INSULIN

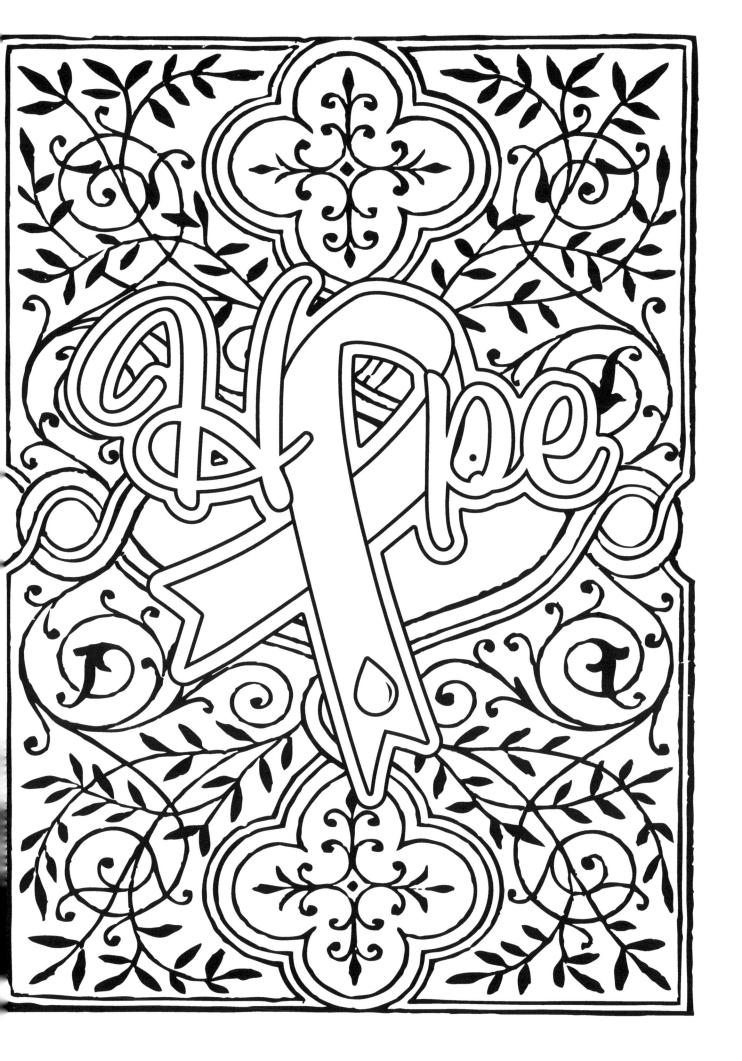

HOPE

A ZOMBIE ATE MY

PANCREAS

A ZOMBIE ATE MY PANCREAS

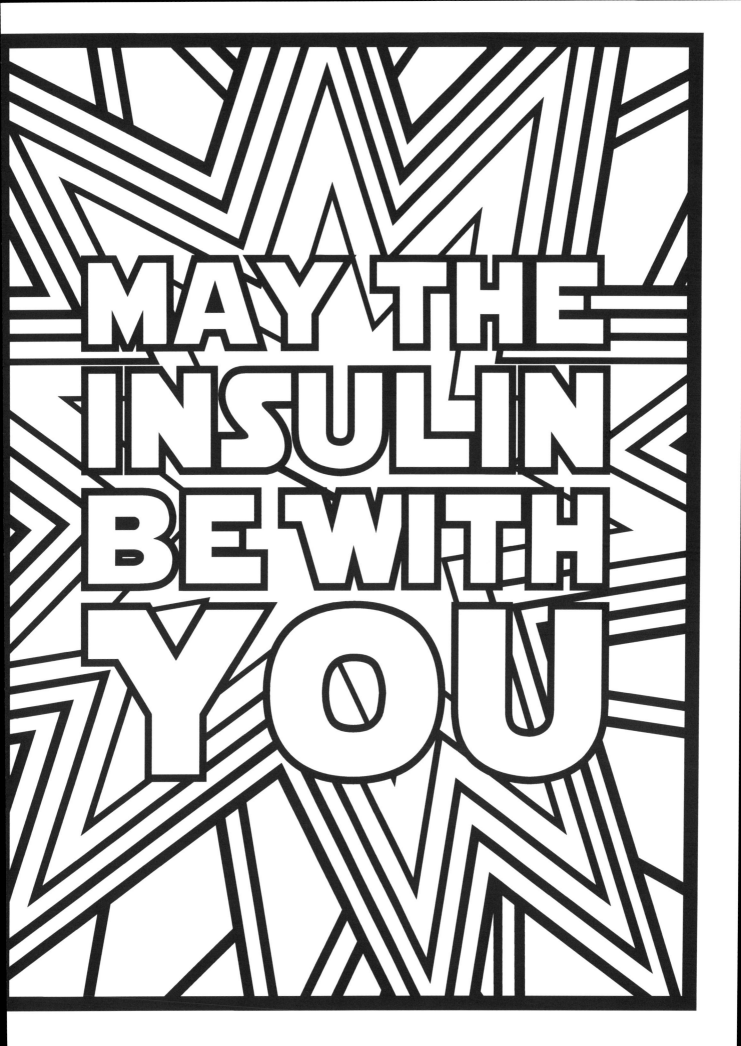

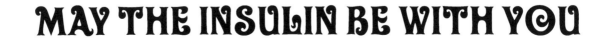

MAY THE INSULIN BE WITH YOU

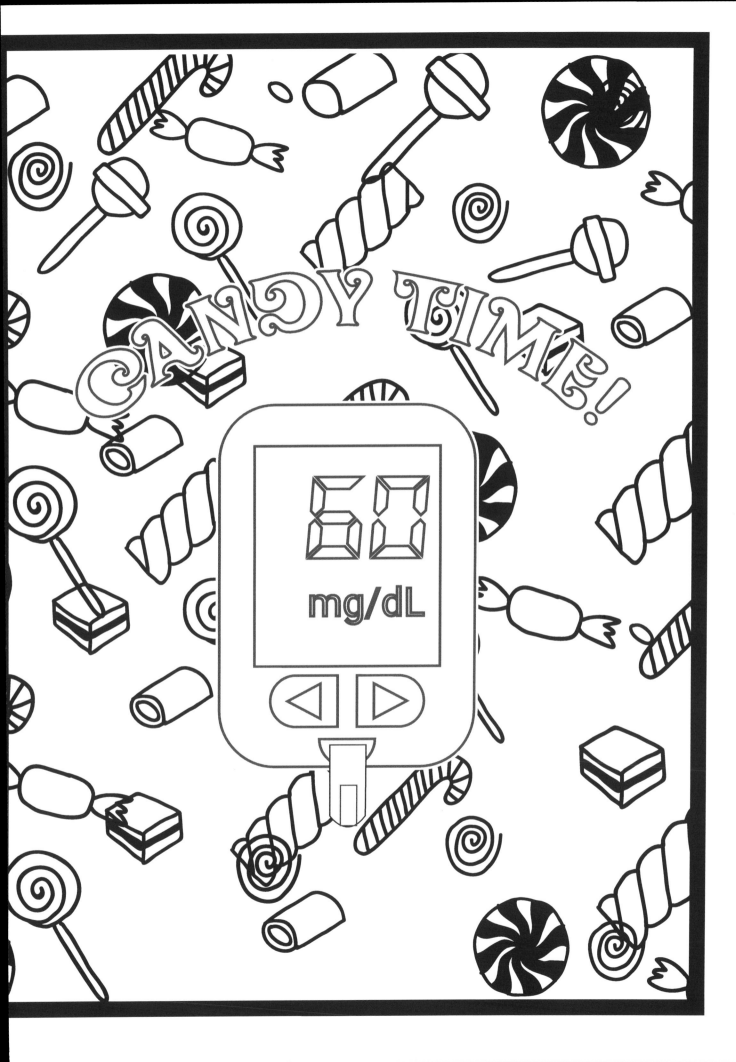

CANDY TIME

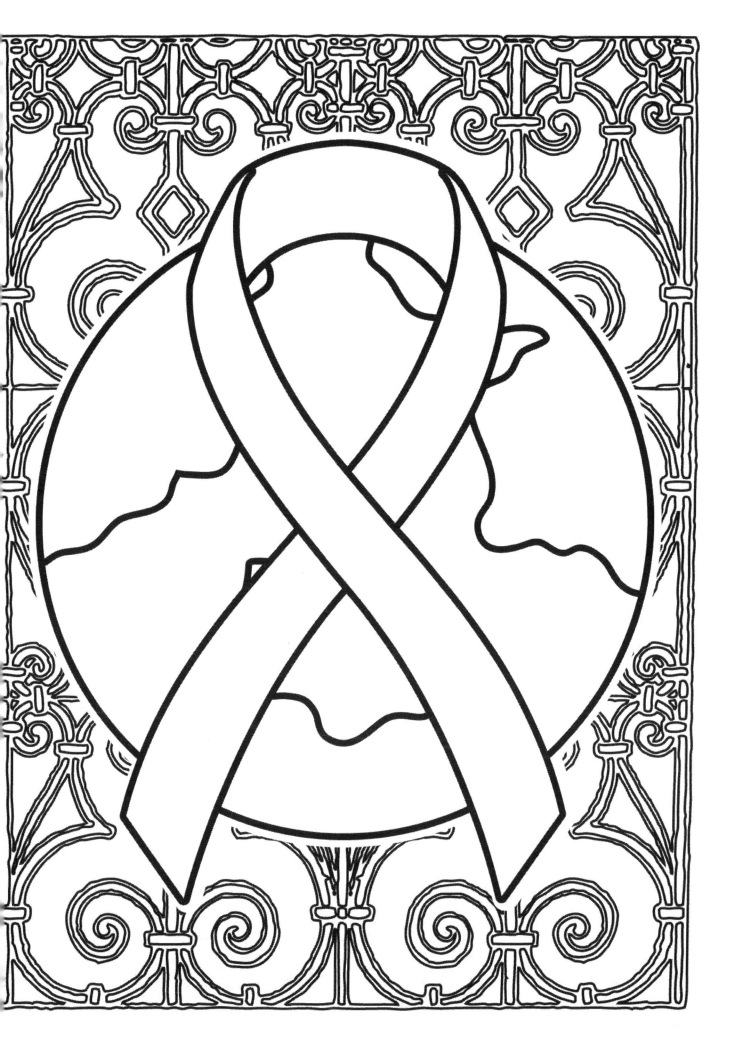

WORLD AWARENESS

WILL BOLUS

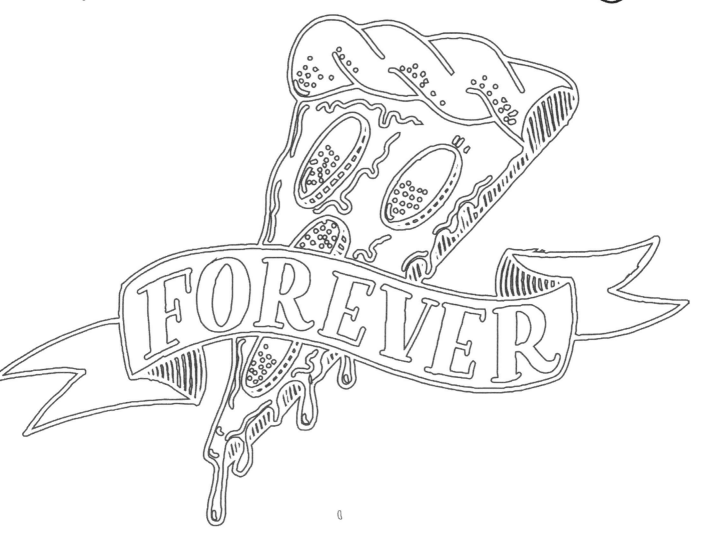

FOR PIZZA

WILL BOLUS FOR PIZZA

Just Give Me The Dang Cupcake and Educate Yourself!

JUST GIVE ME THE DANG CUPCAKE

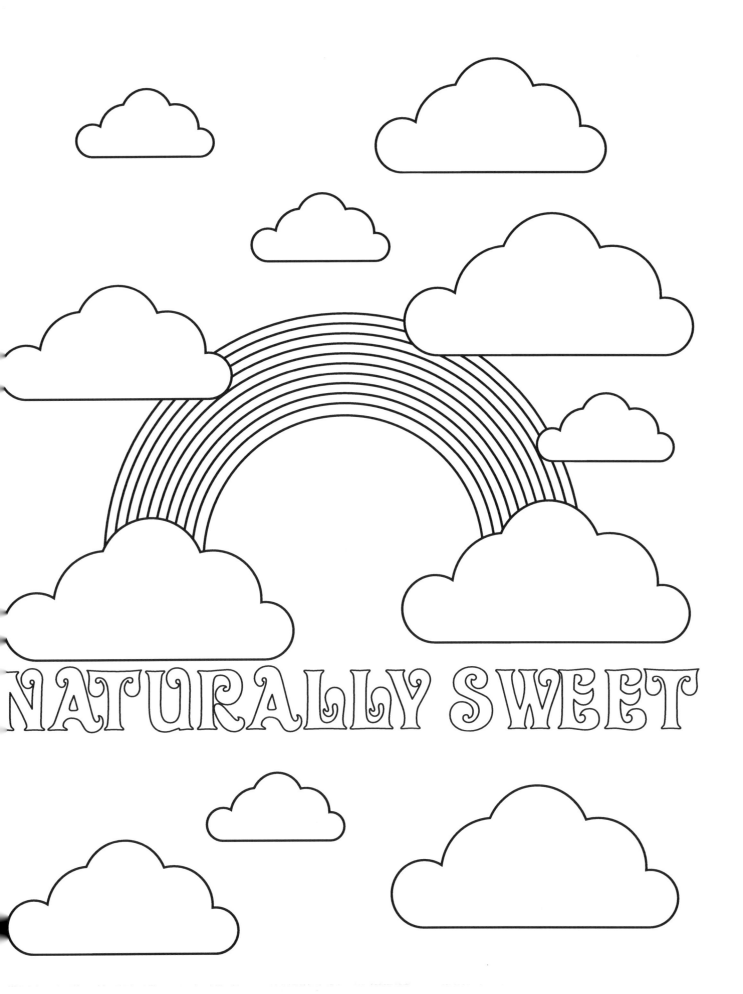

NATURALLY SWEET

NATURALLY SWEET

Made in the USA
Las Vegas, NV
14 January 2025

16364971R00024